CW00404051

The 1x1 Low Carb Cookbook for Beginners

A Complete LC-Guide - Quick and Mouth-Watering Recipes for Everyday Enjoyment incl. 7 Days Meal Plan

Matthew Hollandar

Copyright © [2022] [Matthew Hollandar]

All rights reserved

All rights for this book here presented belong exclusively to the author. Usage or reproduction of the text is forbidden and requires a clear consent of the author in case of expectations.

ISBN - 9798781952137

Table of Contents

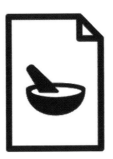

Matthew Hollandar

Section One: Introduction to a low-carb life

Welcome to your new low carb lifestyle! You're taking the plunge into the exciting world of new ingredients, health benefits, and of course, a big lifestyle change! Making any big change like this one can be difficult, confusing or even intimidating, but don't worry. We're here to help. We've broken down a handy introduction for you to help get started. In this book you'll be able to find some things to be aware of when embarking on a low carb journey, some tips to help you get started, and of course a list of recipes for you to try out.

Benefits to a low carb lifestyle

There are a lot of benefits that you can enjoy when going low carb! Here we'll go through a handful for you.

It's flexible!

Oftentimes when we start a diet, we find that it's all about rules. You're restricted to a certain number of calories, or a limited number of food groups, without proper swaps available to make the meals enjoyable. If you've gone through this and come out the other side feeling disheartened then don't worry, because you aren't alone.

Luckily, a low carb lifestyle doesn't have those same restrictions. You don't have to follow a strict calorie guideline, and there are no dietary restrictions that you *need* to follow (except that your meals should be low in carbohydrates of course!) This means that you can adapt a low carb recipe for your individual dietary requirements. Anyone can lead a low carb life, whether you're vegan, gluten intolerant, or suffer with food allergies.

Steady energy levels

Have you gone through the problem of the late afternoon energy crash? Almost all of us have at some point – we stock up on a nice healthy lunch in the hopes that it'll carry us through until dinner, but after only a couple of hours we feel our energy levels crash. You might feel headachy, lethargic, or even start getting the shakes.

Well, that's because our bodies burn through carbohydrates much faster than they do with fats or proteins, so you're likely to get hungry much faster when eating a high-carb diet. When you replace those carbs with something else (as we're going to show you through this book), you might find that your energy levels don't spike and crash in the way that they do on a carb-intensive diet.

A low carb diet can help you to lose weight

Although it isn't the only reason to try a low carb diet, many people have been known to use it for its weight loss benefits. When you cut down on the carbs, your insulin levels remain steadier, meaning that you're less likely to feel those urgent pangs of hunger that we all get a few hours after eating. Also, when you cut down on carbs, you'll usually switch them out for foods that are high in fat and protein, which have the benefit of keeping you feeling full for longer!

Potential Side effects

As with any new diet, when you switch to a low carb lifestyle you might encounter a few side effects. If you aren't prepared for these, they might seem a little intimidating at first, but we're here to explain some of the most common and give you a few ways to mitigate the effects.

Whenever you are undertaking a new diet of any kind, you should always seek the advice of a medical professional, especially if you have any kind of underlying medical condition. This is because of the strain a new diet can put on your body.

The 'Keto Flu'

The so called 'Keto flu' can happen in the first few days or weeks of a low carb lifestyle. During the first few days after you make the transition to a low carb diet, you may experience headaches, brain fog, lethargy, or even some muscle cramps.

While we don't know exactly why this happens, some people think that it might be in part due to the loss of water and minerals in your body. One way to help alleviate these symptoms is to make sure you drink plenty or water with added electrolytes to balance your sodium levels.

Constipation or diarrhea

As with any other new diet, when you make the change to a low carb lifestyle you might experience some digestive issues one way or the other. These problems are temporary, and your symptoms can be alleviated naturally. If you experience diarrhea, we recommend drinking plenty of water to recoup lost fluids. On the other hand, if you experience constipation after transitioning to a low carb lifestyle, it might be due to lower-than-normal fiber levels in your diet. If this is the case, we recommend eating some high fiber vegetables to help.

General issues

In the first few days or weeks after you make the change to a low carb diet, you might notice a general sense of lethargy, particularly if you're an athlete. It's common to notice decreased performance levels in the first few weeks after you change your diet, but this is normal and importantly, it's *temporary*. There's no need to worry if you're experiencing this, and some have even reported that once their bodies adjust, they actually experience better performance levels than they did before they made the change.

The reason behind this dip in performance levels is because your body is adjusting to how and where it gets its energy. Where it ordinarily gets it energy from your carbohydrate stores, when you change to a low-car diet your body will have to work to draw from your fat stores. Until it adapts to this change, you might notice that you're struggling to perform the way that you once did, but don't worry too much. In no time at all you'll be back to your old self.

Important Note

If you experience any underlying health conditions, then you should consult a medical professional before making any serious changes to your diet or lifestyle. Any big dietary changes can put strain on your organs, so it's best to seek the advice of a doctor if you think you might be at increased risk to any of these side effects.

Foods to avoid on a low carb diet

When starting a new low-carb diet, you may struggle at first to be certain of the foods that you can and cannot eat. To help you out a little bit, we've made up a list of foods you should steer clear of, and some other foods that you should make an effort to include in your new diet.

- Grains like bread, pasta, rice and oats
  - ☐ These foods are all famously high in carbs, and this is something that's especially true when it comes to white bread, pasta and rice. These are known as *refined carbs*, and can spike your blood sugar levels
  - ☐ This goes for gluten free swaps as well, as many of them still use grains. While it isn't true for **all** gluten free options, you can't guarantee that something is low carb just because it's gluten free

- Vegetables that grow below ground
  - ☐ Potatoes and sweet potatoes fall into this category as they are both very starchy and high in carbohydrates. Other foods that you might not initially think would fall into the 'high-carb' category include carrots, beets and onions.

- Natural sugars: honey, maple syrup
  - ☐ While natural sugars might be better for you than refined sugars, if you're starting a low-carb diet you should avoid them. Honey and maple syrup are both very high in carbs.

- Certain fruits
  - ☐ Some fruits are surprisingly high in carbohydrates, like bananas and mangos. Eating a little of these should push you over your daily carb intake, but you should be careful about the amount you consume per day.
    - Bananas are particularly high in carbs, coming in at more than 22 grams of carbs per half a cup
    - Other fruits that are particularly high in carbohydrates include cherries, plums, mango and grapes.

- Beer
  - ☐ If you're trying to live a healthier lifestyle, it's a good idea to limit your alcohol intake anyway, but beer can be particularly problematic for those of us undertaking a low-carb lifestyle
  - ☐ Some of you may have already heard the phrase 'there's a loaf of bread in a can of beer', and that's due in part to the nutritional content of the drink
  - ☐ One normal serving of beer can contain around 13 grams of carbs, which can make it hard to stick within a low-carb lifestyle

Matthew Hollandar

- Soft drinks
  - ☐ Due to the high-sugar nature of soft drinks, these are a good idea to cut from your diet when going low-carb
  - ☐ A can of regular coke contains 35g of carbs, and a full-sized bottle contains a huge 159g of carbs!
  - ☐ Luckily for you, if you have a sweet tooth and love soft drinks, we have a swap for you in the next section that might help keep your cravings at bay

- Low fat swaps
  - ☐ People of a certain age might well still believe that low fat options for certain foods like mayonnaise and yoghurts

Foods you should consider including

Now that we've given you a long list of foods to avoid or cut down on during your time on a low carb diet, you might be wondering if there's anything you actually *can* eat! Don't worry, for anyone who's worried about this we have a list of foods that you should consider including or eating more of.

- Lean meats, fish and eggs
  - All of these foods are great options for those of us on low carb diets. They're high in protein, low in carbohydrates, and often a great source of micronutrients. Fish, for example, is a great source of omega 3, and all meat products are good ways to make sure you get your B12 fill for the day

- Cruciferous vegetables
  - This means leafy greens! Kale, broccoli, Brussel sprouts and cabbage are all low in calories and carbs, making them a great option to bulk out your low carb meals if they're looking a little lackluster
  - In fact, most vegetables that grow above ground are low in carbohydrates, making them great options for low carb foodies
    - Asparagus, zucchini, eggplant and tomatoes are all examples of delicious low carb vegetables which are easy to add to a meal in a variety of different ways!

- Nuts and seeds
  - ☐ Nuts and seeds are all phenomenal additions to any low carb diet. Low in carbs but high in proteins and fats, these make great additions or garnishes to your meal
  - ☐ Alternatively, they can be enjoyed on their own as a healthy, filling snack
  - ☐ Due to their high protein, high fiber and high fat nature, both nuts and seeds can help to keep you fuller for longer, which is great if you're also trying to cut back on calories during your low carb journey
  - ☐ Nut butters are also great options to include in your low carb diet but be careful when choosing the right one. Make sure you check the ingredients list and go for an all-natural brand that doesn't add sweeteners. (Many of the natural nut butters are also palm-oil free, which is a bonus!)

- Some fruits
  - ☐ While we warned you off some of the higher-carb fruits that you'd find on a weekly shop, there are some you can enjoy for a naturally sweet addition to your diet.
  - ☐ Berries, for example, can be low in carbs compared to bananas or grapes
    - Blackberries and raspberries come in at 5 net grams of carbs per 100g
    - Strawberries come in at 6 net grams of carbs per 100g

- Be careful when eating berries though, as it can be quite easy to accidentally go over your recommended daily carb intake by grazing on them throughout the day. We recommend weighing out your fruit into a bowl to make sure you don't accidentally go over your limit!

- Beer
  - I know, I know! We *just* told you that beer is something to be avoided on a low carb diet. But if you're someone who likes to relax with a cold beer in hand at the end of the day, (and can't see yourself giving it up for the sake of the diet), then you're in luck. There are plenty of low carb beer brands out there just waiting to be tried!

- Spirits and Wine
  - Alternatively, if you're on the hunt for an alcoholic drink to help wind down at the end of a long day, you might want to look at switch from beer to spirits or wine
  - While beers are usually notoriously high in carbs, wine is relatively low, and spirits have no carbs at all
  - Of course, these should still be drunk in moderation!

Matthew Hollandar

- Baking ingredients
    - ☐ Just because you're going low carb, doesn't mean you need to give up your passion for baking! While typical baked goods are usually high in refined sugars and carbs, there are some swaps you can make easily
    - ☐ Coconut or almond flour are great alternatives to regular flour and are much lower in carbs (plus they're both glutens free!)
    - ☐ Sugar-free sweeteners like stevia can be found in granulated forms (great to dissolve in your morning tea or coffee), or in liquid forms! The best part is, they taste delicious and can easily be added to your baking

Tips to help you begin your low carb lifestyle

Making a big change to your diet or lifestyle can be difficult, and we know that. To make the adjustment a little easier for you, we've compiled a list of tips to make the transition a little easier for you.

Start with small adjustments

Overhauling your diet in a big way (like you might have to do if you choose to go low carb) can be difficult. One way to make things a little easier for yourself is to make small adjustments each day, easing yourself into your new diet and lifestyle. Some people find that jumping into a diet headfirst can be difficult and overwhelming, and this can be disheartening.

Unfortunately, the harder we find a new diet, the more likely we are to turn away from it and go back to our old eating habits. Luckily though, even a big diet change like a low carb diet doesn't have to be hard. Taking things slowly to build yourself up to a low carb lifestyle can make the diet much easier on yourself. We recommend looking through the list of foods to avoid on a low carb diet and slowly going through it, excluding a few more things each week.

Cook from scratch

We all low a good take away or meal out with friends. Unfortunately, when your food is prepared for you, it's hard to know exactly what goes into it, and even when restaurants include the nutritional information for you, you can't be certain that you're going to be able to stick to your diet. Pre-prepared food that you can find in your local supermarket will often give you the same problems.

The easiest way to know exactly what is in each meal you're eating is to make your own food as often as possible. Not only will your food be healthier, but most of the time home-cooked food is actually cheaper than what you'd find in a restaurant.

Of course, there is one common problem that might make this a little more difficult – finding the time to actually cook all your own meals. That brings us to our next tip:

Meal prep

Meal prepping is a great way to make sure you're sorted for meals throughout the week. There is a myriad of benefits to meal-prepping that make a lot of people die-hard fans of it, and here are just a few:

- ☐ It's faster! Cooking a big batch of food in one night and dividing it up for dinner over 3 or 4 nights means that you'll have a healthy meal waiting for you when you get home from work and don't feel like cooking.
- ☐ There's less waste! This is especially true for those of us who are just cooking for 1 or 2 people. You might find that a recipe

yields you far more servings than you can finish in one sitting. Rather than struggling to find a way to get rid of this excess food, it can make a quick meal later in the week.

Buddy up

Dieting is especially hard when you do it alone. One way to mitigate this is to find one of your friends who's also interested in a low carb lifestyle and do it together! Not only is it more fun to do something with a friend, but you'll have the added motivation and accountability from doing it with a friend.

Alternatively, if you don't have a friend who's interested in the low-carb lifestyle, then take to the internet! You can find a lot of online communities around the world filled with people who, like you, are undertaking a low carb diet.

And last of all...

When you're starting a new diet of any kind, the hardest thing to figure out is exactly what you're going to eat. After all, we've given you a list of foods to include and avoid, but you're probably wondering exactly what you can do with them! That's why we've compiled some of our personal favorite recipes for you to help you get started on your journey. Even if you don't consider yourself to be much of a chef, don't panic. These recipes are quick, easy, and most importantly – delicious!

Section Two: Recipes

Breakfast Recipes

Low Carb Pancakes

Serves: 4 people (2 pancakes each)

Prep Time: 3 Minutes | Cook Time: 12 Minutes | Total Time: 15 Minutes

Calories: 146 | Net Carbs: 1.6g | Protein: 6.5g | Fat: 11g | Fiber: 1.8g

Ingredients:

- 1 tbsp powdered sweetener (optional)
- 1 tsp baking powder
- 1 tsp vanilla extract
- ¼ cup (38g) coconut flour
- 2 tbsp butter (melted)
- 3 large eggs
- 6 tbsp (984ml) coconut milk (unsweetened)
- Small amount of melted butter to grease pan

Matthew Hollandar

Instructions:

1. In a small bowl, beat the eggs with a whisk until it begins to froth

2. Add the rest of the ingredients and continue to beat until a smooth (but thick) batter forms

3. Melt the butter in a frying pan or a skillet over a low – medium heat

4. Once the pan has warmed, spoon 2 tbsp of batter per pancake into the pan, and use the back of the spoon to spread and flatten them

5. Fry the pancakes on a medium low heat, until bubbles form across the top (be sure not to move them while you wait, or they may not cook properly)

6. Flip the pancakes and cook for another minute, then serve

Low Carb Breakfast Omelet

Serves: 1 person

Prep Time: 5 Minutes | Cook Time: 10 Minutes | Total Time: 15 Minutes

Calories: 552 | Net Carbs: 3g | Protein: 30g | Fat: 46g | Fiber: 2g

Ingredients:

- 1 pinch of salt
- 1 tbsp chives (chopped)
- 1 tsp olive oil
- ¼ cup (32g) cheddar cheese (shredded)
- ¼ cup (55g) of bacon (diced)
- 2 large eggs
- 4 small white capped mushrooms (sliced)

Instructions:

1. Pre-heat a non-stick frying pan on a high heat

2. While the pan heats, whisk the eggs and salt together in a small bowl

3. Sauté the bacon and mushrooms in the pan – we like to make sure the bacon is nice and crispy here!

4. Set aside the ingredients and clean the pan

5. Add oil to the frying pan or skillet and warm over a medium heat

6. Add the whisked egg and tilt the pan from side to side so that the mixture covers the entire pan

7. Wait until the mixture has thickened and set, and then add the rest of your ingredients back in on top of the egg. (Mushrooms, bacon, cheese and chives)

8. Cook until the cheese starts to melt, and then gently fold your omelet in half using a spatula

9. Serve and enjoy while still hot!

Tofu Scramble

Serves: 2 people

Prep Time: 10 Minutes | Cook Time: 10 Minutes | Total Time | 20 Minutes

Calories: 175 | Net Carbs: 8g | Protein: 14g | Fat: 20g | Fiber: 4g

Ingredients:

- 1 brown onion (diced)
- 1 pinch of salt
- ½ cup (64g) red bell pepper (chopped)
- ½ cup (64g) zucchini (chopped)
- ½ tsp garlic powder
- ½ tsp turmeric
- 1½ tbsp nutritional yeast
- 2 tbsp avocado oil, coconut oil or butter
- 8oz (226g) pack of extra firm tofu
- Paprika to taste

Instructions:

1. Press the tofu between two sheets of kitchen towel to gently squeeze leftover moisture from it. Place a weight on top (like a plate, chopping board or frying pan) in order to press a little extra moisture from it

2. Warm a frying pan over a medium heat, and grease with oil or butter of choice

3. Sauté the vegetables until softened

4. Using a fork, crumble the tofu until it resembles scrambled eggs

5. Add to the pan, and cook over a medium high heat, stirring consistently for 3-4 minutes

6. Season to taste using the last of your ingredients, and cook for 1 extra minute

7. Serve and enjoy!

Low Carb Granola Mix

Serves: 14 people

Prep Time: 10 Minutes | Cook Time: 30 Minutes | Total Time: 40 Minutes

Calories: 310 | Net Carbs: 4.3 | Protein: 9.5g | Fat: 27.1g | Fiber: 4g

Ingredients:

- 1 ½ cup (150g) pecans

- 1 ½ cup (215g) almonds

- 1 cup (115g) shredded coconut

- 1/3 cup (60g) granulated sweetener

- 1/3 cup (90g) sugar free peanut butter

- ¼ cup (35g) sunflower seeds

- ¼ cup (60g) butter (can be substituted for a dairy free alternative, or coconut oil)

- ¼ cup (60ml) water

Matthew Hollandar

Instructions:

1. Preheat oven to 300 degrees F (150 degrees C)

2. Line a rimmed baking sheet with baking paper

3. Process the almonds and pecans in a food processor. Blitz them until they resemble coarse crumbs (make sure not to make them too fine)

4. Add to a large bowl along with the sunflower seeds, sweetener and shredded coconut

5. Use your microwave to melt the butter and the peanut butter. Be careful to use a microwavable bowl for this. Heat for 30 seconds at first, and from then only use the microwave in increments of 10 seconds to make sure they don't boil or scorch

6. When melted, pour this mixture over the dried ingredients and stir well, before adding the water. The mixture should now be clumping together, and it should be quite thick

7. Spread the mixture out over the baking sheet and press down firmly, flattening it against the baking sheet

8. Bake for 15 minutes before removing from the oven. Stir the mixture and press it down again, before placing back in the oven. Cook for a further 15 minutes

9. Remove from the oven and allow to cool completely until it goes hard. Break up any large pieces before serving

Matthew Hollandar

Low Carb Overnight "Oats"

Serves: 2 people

Prep Time: 5 minutes | Chill Time: 4+ hours | Total Time: 4+ hours

Calories: 284 | Net Carbs: 2.1 | Protein: 11.3g | Fat: 24.7g | Fiber: 2.9

Ingredients:

- 1 Pinch of salt
- 1 tbsp Golden flaxseed
- 1/2tbsp Chia seeds
- ¼ cup (30g) Hemp hearts
- ¼ cup (60ml) heavy cream
- ¼ cup (60ml) unsweetened coconut milk

Instructions:

1. Mix the dried ingredients together in a bowl or mason jar

2. Stir in the cream and milk

3. Cover the bowl or mason jar and leave to chill in the fridge overnight (but if you really can't wait that long, leave for at least 4 hours!)

Ultimate Low Carb Breakfast Hash

Serves: 1 person

Prep Time: 5 Minutes | Cook Time: 20 Minutes | Total Time: 25 Minutes

Calories: 481| Net Carbs: 7.6g | Protein: 26.3g | Fat: 36.5 | Fiber:7.8g

Ingredients:

- 1 ½ cup (160g) Cauliflower (chopped)
- 1 cup spinach (chopped
- 1 tbsp fresh chopped parsley (optional)
- ½ red bell pepper (chopped)
- ½ tsp pepper
- ¼ cup (55g) of bacon (diced)
- 2 large eggs
- 3 spring onion (sliced)
- Half a large avocado (sliced)
- 1 Pinch of salt

Instructions:

1. Preheat a nonstick frying pan or cast-iron skillet over a medium head

2. Add the bacon to the pan and cook until crispy (should take between 3-5 minutes). When cooked to your taste, remove and set aside in a small bowl

3. In the leftover fat from the bacon, cook the cauliflower, pepper and spring onions. Season to taste and cook until the vegetables have softened, stirring occasionally. This should take around 10 minutes

4. Stir in the spinach and cook for around 1 minute, until you can see the leaves starting to wilt

5. Turn the heat down to the lowest setting and use a spoon to make 2 wells in the mixture. Crack 2 eggs, 1 into each of the wells. Season to taste, and then cover with a lid. Cook until the egg whites have set. (This should take around 5 minutes)

6. Sprinkle your fresh herbs and crispy bacon on top and serve with sliced avocado while still warm

Avocado Breakfast scramble

Serves: 1 person

Prep Time: 5 Minutes | Cook Time: 20 Minutes | Total Time: 15 Minutes

Calories: 815 | Net Carbs: 8g | Protein: 40g | Fat: 60g | Fiber: 8g

Ingredients:

- ½ avocado (sliced)
- ½ cup (110g) cheddar cheese (shredded)
- ¼ cup (40g) Pico de Gallo (optional, to top the recipe)
- 2 large eggs
- 3 slices of bacon (chopped)
- Salt and pepper (optional, to taste)

Instructions:

1. Preheat a nonstick frying pan or skillet on a medium – high heat. Add the chopped bacon to the pan or skillet and cook until it's crispy

2. Scramble the eggs in a small bowl while the bacon cooks. Add any salt, pepper or other seasoning to the eggs here

3. When the bacon has cooked, set aside in a small bowl. Do not drain any leftover fat from the bacon – we'll use this to cook the eggs!

4. Turn the heat down to a medium – low heat. Pour the eggs into the pan to start cooking them. Stir constantly to scramble them to your desired consistency. The goal here is to never let the eggs settle for too long – the longer the eggs settle on the base of the pan, the larger the pieces of scrambled egg will be

5. Once cooked, pour the eggs into a bowl, and then top with shredded cheese, the bacon, and sliced avocado. If you'd like to add the freshness of some Pico de Gallo, add that here!

Lunch Recipes

Avocado chicken Salad with lemon dressing

Serves: 6 people

Prep Time: 15 minutes | Cook Time 15 minutes | Total Time: 30 minutes

Calories: 400 | Net Carbs: 3g | Protein: 19.2g | Fat: 32g | Fiber: 3.g

Ingredients:

- 1 cup (120g) cucumber
- 1 garlic clove (crushed)
- ½ tsp salt
- 14 oz (400g) g pre-cooked chicken (rotisserie chicken works well).
- 2 cups (70g) lettuce (shredded)
- 2 large avocados (cubed)
- 2 tbsp fresh parsley (finely chopped)
- 3 tbsp extra virgin olive oil
- 3 tbsp lemon juice
- 6 oz (170g) bacon (fried and chopped)
- Pepper to taste

Matthew Hollandar

Instructions:

1. Heat a frying pan or skillet on a medium – high heat until crispy. Store in a small bowl in the fridge until needed. Preferably wait until it has cooled completely before using

2. Shred the chicken using two forks, pulling it apart into small pieces

3. Set aside in the fridge in a bowl until needed

4. Make up a lemon dressing to top the salad

   a. Add the lemon juice, olive oil, salt, pepper and crushed garlic to a bowl and whisk until mixed properly. Only do this once you are ready to serve, otherwise the ingredients might separate!

5. In a large bowl, add the chicken, bacon, cucumber, lettuce and cubed avocado and mix together

6. Pour the lemon dressing over the top of your salad and mix everything again. Sprinkle with parsley and serve

Low Carb lettuce tacos

Serves: 4 people

Prep Time: 30 Minutes | Cook Time 15 Minutes | Total Time: 45 minutes

Calories: 320 | Net Carbs: 9.8g | Protein: 29g | Fat: 18.1g | Fiber: 2.2g

Ingredients:

For the chicken

- 1 tbsp olive oil
- 1lb (600g) boneless, skinless chicken breast
- 2 cloves of garlic (minced or finely chopped)
- 2 tbsp taco seasoning

For the tacos

- 1 large avocado (chopped)
- 1 large tomato (diced)
- ¼ cup (35g) onion (diced)
- 8 leaves romaine lettuce (rinsed and dried) (2 leaves per person)

Matthew Hollandar

For the coriander sauce

- 1 glove garlic (minced)
- 1 jalapeno pepper (optional)
- 1 pinch of salt
- ½ cup (120g) Greek yoghurt (this can be substituted for sour cream or mayonnaise)
- ½ cup (4g) loosely packed coriander (cilantro)
- 2 tbsp olive oil
- The juice of ½ a lime

Instructions:

1. Cook the chicken

   a. Add the chicken, olive oil, garlic and taco seasoning to a bowl or zip lock bag. If using a bowl, cover properly and store in the fridge to marinade. Ideally this would be done overnight to really seal the flavors in, but 30 minutes will do if you're in a rush

   b. Preheat a nonstick pan or skillet on a medium – high heat

   c. Once marinaded, remove the chicken from the bag and place on the pan. Cook the chicken until it is white throughout, which should take about 10 minutes on each side. Cooking time depends on the thickness of the chicken. To check that it's cooked through, slice through the middle of the thickest piece of chicken and pull apart gently using a fork

2. Make the cilantro sauce

    a. Place the olive oil, jalapeno, lime juice, salt, coriander, yoghurt and garlic into a food processor and blitz until creamy. Simple!

3. Assemble the tacos

    a. Roughly chop the chicken into cubes, and layer it into a lettuce leaf alone with tomatoes, avocado and onion. Drizzle with the coriander sauce you made earlier and enjoy

Cauliflower Fried Rice

Serves: 6 people

Prep Time: 5 Minutes | Cook Time: 10 Minutes | Total Time: 15 Minutes

Calories: 109 | Net Carbs: 4.9g | Protein: 5.4g | Fat: 6.6g | Fiber: 3.5g

Ingredients:

- 1 large cauliflower
- ½ green bell pepper (finely chopped)
- ½ red bell pepper (finely chopped)
- 2 large eggs (whisked)
- 2 tbsp butter, ghee or oil of choice (preferably coconut)
- 2 tbsp sesame oil
- 2 tbsp soy sauce (alternatively substitute for tamari)
- 2.5 tbsp fresh ginger (grated)
- 3 spring onions (finely chopped)
- 4 garlic cloves (minced roughly)
- Salt and pepper (to taste)

Instructions:

1. Roughly chop the cauliflower and add the florets into a food processor, blitzing until it resembles rice. Alternatively, use the larger holes of a box grater to grate the cauliflower into a rice like consistency

2. Warm a frying pan or wok over a medium – high heat. Melt the butter, ghee or oil and stir fry the peppers, ginger, garlic and the whites of the spring onions. Fry for 3 minutes until softened, stirring regularly

3. Add the cauliflower to the pan and fry for 3 minutes, stirring consistently. After 3 minutes, push the mix to one side of the pan

4. Whisk the eggs and season with salt and pepper according to your own taste. Add to the side of the pan not taken up by the cauliflower rice and scramble them until they reach a desired texture

5. Once cooked, mix the eggs with the cauliflower rice. Drizzle sesame oil over the top and serve with the greens of the onions

Matthew Hollandar

Stuffed Avocados

Serves: 4 people

Prep Time: 5 minutes | Cook Time: 10 minutes | Total Time: 15 minutes

Calories: 334 | Net Carbs: 6.4g | Protein: 20.3g | Fat: 25.2g | Fiber: 3.4g

Ingredients:

- 1 pre-cooked chicken breast (shredded)

- ¼ cup (30g) Parmesan cheese (grated)

- 2 large avocadoes (halved and pitted)

- 2 oz (60g) cream cheese (softened)

- 2 tbsp tomatoes (chopped)

- Salt, pepper and cayenne pepper to taste

Instructions:

1. Preheat your oven to 400 degrees F (200 degrees C)

2. Scoop out a little of the flesh of the avocado to make a mid-sized well

3. Add the chicken, cream cheese, tomatoes and seasoning to the well in the avocadoes, and top with cheese

4. Place in the preheated oven and bake until cheese has melted fully (about 10 minutes)

Broccoli Salad

Serves: 4 people

Prep Time: 15 minutes | Cook Time: 10 minutes | Total Time: 25 minutes

Calories: 502 | Net Carbs: 9g | Protein: 17g | Fat: 44g | Fiber: 4g

Ingredients:

- 1 cup (110g) cheddar cheese (shredded
- 1 packet of sweetener
- 1/3 cup (40g) walnuts (chopped)
- ½ cup (60g) red onion (diced)
- ¼ cup (30g) mayonnaise
- ¼ cup (30g) sour cream
- ¼ cup (30g) sunflower seeds
- 2 tbsp apple cider vinegar
- 4 cups of broccoli florets (520g) (roughly chopped)
- 6 slices bacon

Instructions:

1. Warm a pan or skillet over a high heat and cook the bacon until very crispy. Crumble and leave in a small bowl and set aside in the fridge until needed. Pour any of the leftover bacon fat into a separate bowl

2. Mix the sour cream, mayonnaise, apple cider vinegar and sweetener in with the leftover bacon fat

3. In a large mixing bowl, toss together the bacon, sunflower seeds, walnut, onion, broccoli and cheese

4. Pour the dressing over the top of the mixture and leave to settle for 10 minutes before serving

Tuna Salad

Serves: 2 people

Prep Time: 10 minutes | Cook Time: 10 minutes | Total Time: 20 minutes

Calories: 614 | Net Carbs: 6g | Protein: 33g | Fat: 50g | Fiber: 4g

Ingredients:

- 1 1/4 (160g) cups celery stalks
- 1 ¼ cups (160g) tuna in olive oil
- ½ a lemon (juiced)
- ¼ cup (30g) mayonnaise
- 1tsp Dijon mustard
- 2 spring onions
- 2 tbsp olive oil
- 4 eggs
- 4 oz (115g) cherry tomatoes
- 6 oz (170g) romaine lettuce
- Salt and pepper, to taste

Instructions:

1. Chop the celery and spring onions finely and add to a large mixing bowl. Also add the tuna, mayonnaise and mustard. Stir well to combine and season with salt and pepper according to taste. Put in fridge until needed

2. Add the eggs to a saucepan of boiling water and leave to simmer for 5-10 minutes, depending on how you like your eggs. If you prefer soft-medium, cook for closer to 5 minutes. If you prefer eggs hardboiled, cook for 10 minutes

3. As soon as the eggs are done, place in ice-cold water to make them easier to peel. Peel the shell off and cut the eggs into halves, quarters or smaller segments (depending on your preference)

4. Place the eggs and tuna on a bed of romaine lettuce. Add tomatoes and drizzle olive oil on top to garnish before serving

Stir Fry Chicken

Serves: 4

Prep Time: 10 minutes | Cook Time: 20 minutes | Total Time: 30 minutes

Calories: 310 | Net Carbs: 5g | Protein: 43g | Fat: 46g | Fiber: 2g

Ingredients:

For the stir-fried chicken

- 1 1/3 lbs (800g) boneless chicken thighs, thinly sliced
- 1 tsp black pepper
- 1 tsp garlic powder
- 10 oz (280g) broccoli (chopped into small pieces)
- 2 tbsp olive oil
- 2 tbsp tamari soy sauce

For the spicy mayonnaise

- 1 tsp garlic powder
- 2 tbsp sugar free hot sauce
- ¾ cup (180ml) mayonnaise

Instructions:

1. To make the mayonnaise, add the hot sauce, mayonnaise and garlic powder to a small bowl and stir well. Set this aside in the fridge to keep cool until needed at the end

2. Warm a frying pan or a wok over a medium to high heat. Add the chicken, garlic and pepper to the pan and stir fry until the chicken turns golden brown. Be sure to keep moving the ingredients around the pan so that nothing burns. This is vital to remember when cooking on a high heat!

3. Add the broccoli and tamari soy sauce. Stir the ingredients until the broccoli is tender, but be sure not to overcook it, because it will lose the crispness

4. Serve immediately, with the spicy mayonnaise as a side (or drizzled over the top!)

Low Carb Quesadilla

Serves: 2 people

Prep Time: 15 minutes | Cook Time: 25 Minutes | Total Time: 40 minutes

Calories: 599 | Net Carbs: 5.4g | Protein: 52.7g | Fat: 40g | Fiber: 1g

Ingredients:

- 1 ½ (190g) cup Cheddar cheese (grated)
- 1 ½ cup (190g) Mozzarella cheese (shredded)
- 1 cup (130g) pre-cooked chicken (chopped)
- 1/3 cup (40g) red bell pepper (diced)
- 1/8 cup (15g) spring onion (finely chopped)
- ¼ cup (30g) tomato (diced)

Instructions:

1. Pre-heat your oven to 400 degrees F (200 degrees C) and cover a pizza pan with baking paper

2. Miz the cheese together in a bowl, and then spread across the paper

3. Bake the cheese for 5 minutes, until it forms a shell. Be careful not to over-cook it, because if you do then it won't fold into a quesadilla

4. Place the chicken, peppers, tomato and onion over one half of the cheese shell. Carefully fold the other half of the cheese shell over the chicken and vegetable mixture and press down firmly

5. Return to the oven and bake for another 5 minutes, serve immediately

Dinner Recipes

Keto Chicken Soup

Serves: 4 people

Prep Time: 10 Minutes | Cook Time: 30 Minutes | Total Time: 40 Minutes

Calories: 286 | Net Carbs: 7.5g | Protein: 29g | Fat: 14.9 | Fiber: 2.7

Ingredients:

- 1 brown onion (finely chopped)
- 1 cup (50g) chopped kale
- 1 garlic clove (minced)
- 1 regular leek (chopped)
- 1 tbsp butter (alternatively substitute with extra virgin olive oil
- 1 tbsp thyme leaves (finely chopped)
- 1.5 ltr chicken stock
- 10 oz (300g) cooked chicken
- 2 bay leaves
- 2 medium carrots (peeled and roughly chopped)
- 3 stalks of celery (chopped)
- 8g fresh parsley
- Salt and pepper to taste

Instructions:

1. Heat the butter or oil in a soup pot on a medium heat. Sauté the carrots, leek and celery with the thyme and about half the parsley. Cook until they have softened, which should take around 5 minutes

2. Add the stock, bay leaves and seasoning, and bring to the boil. Reduce the heat to low and place a lid on the soup pot. Leave to simmer for 15 minutes

3. Divide the soup in half, leaving one half in the pot. Remove the bay leaves as well. Using a hand blender, pulse the soup to thicken it

4. Add the rest of the soup mixture, as well as the cooked chicken and kale. Simmer until the chicken has been heated through, and then serve, topped with the last of the fresh parsley

Keto Pizza

Serves: 8 people

Prep Time: 10 minutes | Cook Time: 15 minutes | Total Time: 20 minutes

Calories: 255 | Net Carbs: 5g | Protein: 14g | Fat: 19g | Fiber: 2g

Ingredients:

- 1 cup almond flour
- 1 large egg
- 1 tsp baking powder
- 1tsp garlic powder
- 2 cups Mozzarella cheese (shredded)
- 2 tbsp cream cheese
- Fresh mozzarella (as a topping)
- Italian dried herbs
- Sugar free tomato sauce

Instructions:

1. Preheat your oven to 450 degrees F (230 degrees C)

2. In a microwavable bowl, add the shredded mozzarella and cream cheese, and microwave for 30 seconds

3. Remove from microwave and add the egg, almond flour, Italian seasoning, garlic and baking powder. Mix well until a dough form

4. Place the dough on a large sheet of baking paper and place another sheet of baking paper on top. Using a rolling pin, flatten the dough into a sheet about ¼ inch thick. Remove the top layer of baking paper

5. Transfer the pizza base onto a baking sheet and back for 10 minutes

6. Remove the pizza base from the oven, and load with toppings however you'd prefer (this is where the sugar free tomato sauce and fresh mozzarella come in!)

7. Bake for another 8 minutes until the cheese is bubbling and serve hot!

Garlic Shrimp

Serves: 4 people

Prep Time: 15 minutes | Cook Time: 10 minutes | Total Time: 25 minutes

Calories: 488 | Net Carbs: 4g | Protein: 30g | Fat: 44g | Fiber: 2g

Ingredients:

- 1 ½ cups heavy cream
- 1 lbs (500g) shrimp
- ½ cup dry white wine
- ½ cup Parmesan (grated)
- 1tbsp extra virgin olive oil
- 2 tbsp butter
- 2 tbsp fresh parsley (chopped)
- 6 cloves garlic (minced)
- Salt and pepper, to taste

Instructions:

1. Heat the olive oil over a high heat. Season the shrimp with a little salt and pepper, and fry for 1-2 minutes on each side. You want to make sure that they are just cooked through and pink. Set aside in a bowl

2. Melt the butter in the same pan used for the shrimp. Sauté the garlic for around 30 seconds to 1 minute and pour in the white wine. Allow to reduce down to about half of the original volume, and scrape any garlic that sticks to the bottom of the pan

3. Reduce heat to low and add the cream. Allow to gently simmer for a few minutes, stirring occasionally. As it simmers, it should start to thicken up. Season with a little more salt and pepper

4. Add the parmesan cheese and allow to simmer for 2-3 more minutes

5. Return the shrimp to the pan and season with parsley. Cook until warmed through and serve hot

Lemon and Garlic Salmon

Serves: 4 people

Prep Time: 10 minutes | Cook Time: 12 minutes | Total Time: 22 minutes

Calories: 589 | Net Carbs: 4g | Protein: 41g | Fat: 44g | Fiber: 3g

Ingredients:

- 1 lemon
- 1 tbsp parsley (finely chopped)
- 1 tsp onion powder
- 1.5lbs salmon, (sliced into 4 fillets)
- ½ cup butter (melted)
- ½ tsp pepper
- 1lbs asparagus (trimmed)
- 3 cloves garlic (minced)
- Pinch of salt

Matthew Hollandar

Instructions:

1. Preheat your oven to 450 degrees F (230 degrees C)

2. Melt the butter in your microwave in 30 second increments. Whisk the butter with the garlic, parsley and onion powder together

3. Line a baking tray with baking paper and lay the fillets on the sheet. Be careful to space them out so the fillets aren't touching

4. Lay the asparagus around the fillets of salmon on the baking sheet, and drizzle the garlic butter over the top

5. Bake for 12-15 minutes, until the salmon is opaque throughout, and squeeze the lemon juice over the top before serving

Zucchini Lasagna

Serves: 6 people

Prep Time: 20 minutes | Cook Time: 40 minutes | Total Time: 60 minutes

Calories: 644 | Net Carbs: 7g | Protein: 34g | Fat: 53g | Fiber: 2g

Ingredients:

- 1 ½ Lbs (500g) ground beef
- 1 brown onion (finely chopped)
- 1 regular zucchini (thinly sliced)
- 1 tbsp dried oregano
- 1 tbsp fried basil
- 1 tsp salt
- ¼ tsp ground black pepper
- 2 tbsp olive oil
- 3 tbsp water
- 4 tbsp tomato paste

For the cheese sauce

- 1 ½ (360 ml) cups heavy cream
- 1 garlic clove (minced)
- 2 cups (260g) cheddar cheese (shredded)

Instructions:

1. Preheat your oven to 400 degrees F (200 degrees C), and set a deep baking dish aside

2. Use a vegetable peeler to thinly slice the zucchini lengthways. Lay the slices on a paper towel and sprinkle lightly with salt. Allow them to rest, and then pat dry with paper towels

3. While the zucchini slices are resting, heat the olive oil on a medium heat, in a large pan or skillet. Sauté the onion and garlic until softened, and then add the ground beef, basil, oregano, salt and pepper. Mix well and cook until the meat has browned

4. Stir in the tomato paste and water until fully mixed with the meat. Reduce the heat to low and allow the mixture to simmer for 10 minutes. Stir occasionally to make sure it cooks through

5. In a separate saucepan, add the garlic, cream and half of the shredded cheese. On a medium heat, bring the mixture to a simmer and allow to melt and thicken. Salt to taste

6. Assemble the lasagna carefully. Spread 1/3 of the meat sauce on the bottom of the baking dish. Cover with a layer of the thin cheese sauce, then cover with zucchini slices. Repeat the layers until all of the ingredients have been used, and then sprinkle with the remaining cheese

7. Bake in the oven for 20 minutes until the cheese is golden. Once cooked, turn off the oven and allow it to rest for 15 minutes

Matthew Hollandar

Keto Burgers

Serves: 4 people

Prep Time: 25 minutes | Cook Time: 15 minutes | Total Time: 40 minutes

Calories: 1000 | Net Carbs: 8g | Protein: 54g | Fat: 82g | Fiber: 5g

Ingredients:

For the burger

- 1 1/2 lbs (650g) ground beef
- 1 cup (110g) cheddar cheese (shredded)
- 2 tbsp butter
- 2 tbsp fresh oregano (finely chopped)
- 2 tsp garlic powder
- 2 tsp onion powder
- 2 tsp paprika powder

For the toppings

- ½ cup (120ml) mayonnaise
- 4 tbsp Dijon mustard
- 4 tbsp jalapenos
- 5 oz (140g) cooked bacon (crumbled)
- 5 oz (140g) lettuce

For the salsa

- 1 large avocado
- 1 tbsp olive oil
- 2 large tomatoes
- 2 spring onions
- 2 tbsp fresh coriander (finely chopped)
- Salt, to taste

Matthew Hollandar

Instructions:

1. Chop up the salsa ingredients finely and stir together well in a small bowl. Set aside in the fridge to keep them chilled until ready to use

2. Mix in the seasoning and half of the cheese with the ground beef. Combine until the spices are thoroughly mixed in with the beef

3. Divide the ground beef into 4 and mold 4 burger patties. Warm a frying pan or skillet on a high heat and fry the burgers. Towards the end of cooking, sprinkle the remainder of the cheese on top

4. Serve with lettuce, mayonnaise, bacon, mustard and homemade salsa

Chicken and Eggplant

Serves: 4

Prep Time: 2+ hours | Cook Time: 35 minutes | Total Time: 2 hours and 35 minutes

Calories: 880 | Net Carbs: 9g | Protein: 44g | Fat: 72g | Fiber: 5g

Ingredients:

For the Tzatziki

- ½ cup (90g) Greek yoghurt

- ¼ cup (60ml) mayonnaise

- 2 cloves garlic (minced)

- 2 oz (55g) cucumber (peeled and shredded)

- Salt and pepper to taste

For the marinade

- 1 ½ tsp salt

- 1 lemon (juiced)

- 1 tbsp dried oregano

- 1/3 cup (80ml) extra virgin olive oil

- ½ tsp ground cinnamon

- ½ tsp ground pepper

- 2 garlic cloves (minced)

- 2 tsp chili flakes (optional)

Chicken, vegetables and cheese

- 14 oz (400g) eggplant (cubed)

- 2 oz (55g) feta cheese (crumbled)

- 2lbs (900g) chicken thighs (with bone and skin)

- 8 cherry tomatoes

Instructions:

1. Preheat your oven to 375 degrees F (200 degrees C). Line a baking sheet with baking paper

2. Combine all ingredients for you marinade in a large bowl. Place the chicken and eggplant into the bowl and coat thoroughly. Allow to chill in the refrigerator for 2+ hours

3. In a large bowl, make the tzatziki. Mix the cucumber, yoghurt, mayonnaise and garlic. Season with salt and pepper to taste and set to one side for later

4. Spread the chicken, eggplant and tomatoes on the baking sheet. Bake in the over for 35 minutes until the skin on the chicken is crispy and it has cooked through

5. Remove the baking tray from the oven and sprinkle the feta cheese on top. Garnish with the tzatziki

Coconut Curry

Serves: 4 people

Prep Time: 15 minutes | Cook Time: 20 minutes | Total Time: 35 minutes

Calories: 291 | Net Carbs: 6g | Protein: 5g | Fat: 28g | Fiber: 2g

Ingredients:

- 1.41 oz (40g) Keto friendly Thai green curry paste

- 16 oz (480ml) coconut cream

- 2.9 oz (80g) button mushrooms

- 3 oz (80g) broccoli

- 3 oz (80g) zucchini

Instructions:

1. On a medium heat, warm the wok or frying pan. Pour about 1/3 of the coconut cream into the wok and allow it to simmer

2. As it begins to bubble, add in the Thai green curry paste and stir it in

3. Add the vegetables and stir into the mixture. Cook until they begin to soften, and then add the rest of the coconut milk on top

Allow to simmer for a further 5 minutes and serve hot – feel free to serve over our cauliflower rice!

Low Carb Sesame Chicken

Serves: 4 people

Prep Time: 15 minutes | Cook Time: 15 minutes | Total Time: 30 minutes

Calories: 338 | Net Carbs: 1.4g | Protein: 53.6g | Fat: 11.2g | Fiber: 1g

Ingredients:

- 1 ½ lbs boneless chicken breast
- 1 tbsp extra virgin olive oil
- 1 tbsp white wine vinegar
- 1.2 tbsp Xanthan gum
- 2 tbsp liquid sweetener
- 2 tsp minced garlic
- 2 tsp minced ginger
- 2 tsp sesame oil
- 3 tbsp soy sauce
- Salt and pepper, to your taste

Instructions:

1. Chop up the chicken into bite sized chunks, and coat in salt and pepper according to your taste

2. Place the chicken pieces into a zip lock bag and sprinkle ½ tbsp Xanthan gum into the bag on the chicken. Close the bag and shake it to fully coat the chicken

3. In a frying pan or skillet, heat 1 tbsp olive oil and 1 tbsp sesame oil over a medium – high heat

4. Cook the chicken pieces in the pan, being careful not to overcrowd the span. If you do, the pieces won't cook properly. If you need to, cook the chicken in 2 batches

5. Cook the chicken for 4 minutes on one side, then flip to the other side to allow the chicken to cook the whole way through

6. While the chicken is cooking in the pan, add the soy sauce, sweetener, ginger paste, garlic, vinegar and oil into a small bowl, and whisk well

7. Pour the sauce over the chicken stir well, before serving – we recommend this with cauliflower rice!

Low Carb Meatloaf

Serves: 8

Prep Time: 15 Minutes | Cook Time: 60 Minutes | Total times: 75 Minutes

Calories: 215 | Net Carbs: 3g | Protein: 17g | Fat: 14g | Fiber: 2g

Ingredients:

- 1 brown onion (finely chopped)
- 1 tbsp dried Italian herbs
- ½ cup (70g) almond flour
- ½ tsp black pepper
- ¼ cup (30g) sugar free ketchup
- ¼ cup (60ml) + tablespoon milk (use any milk of choice)
- 2 large eggs
- 2 tbsp fresh parsley (finely chopped)
- 2 tbsp Worcestershire sauce
- 2 tsp seat salt
- 2lbs ground beef (900g) (choose any ground beef that isn't low fat)
- 3 tbsp sugar free ketchup to glaze meatloaf (optional)

- ¾ cup (90g) keto friendly breadcrumbs
- 4 cloves of garlic (finely chopped)

Instructions:

1. Preheat the oven to 180 degrees C (350 F)

2. Grease a 9x5 inch loaf tin and put to one side for later

3. Combine ground beef, chopped onion and almond flour in a large bowl, before adding the seasonings. Lastly, add the wet ingredients to the bowl and mix well (be careful not to overmix)

4. Transfer the mixture to the loaf pan, and cover with tinfoil to keep the meatloaf moist

5. Bake for 30 minutes before uncovering. If you are using a glaze, you should now spread it across the top of the loaf. Return to the oven and cook for a further 20-45 minutes until cooked through

6. Check that the internal temperature reaches 70 degrees C (160 degrees F). Leave the loaf to rest for 10 minutes before slicing and serving up

Matthew Hollandar

Snacks & Sides

Low Carb Bread Rolls

Serves: 12

Prep Time: 10 minutes | Cook Time: 18 minutes | Total Time: 28 minutes

Calories: 261g | Net Carbs: 4.2g | Protein: 14.4g | Fat: 20.5g | Fiber: 2g

Ingredients:

- 1 ¼ (170g) cups almond flour

- 1 tsp baking soda

- 1/2 tsp salt

- ½ tsp baking powder

- ¼ cup (35g) coconut flour

- ¼ cup (60ml) buttermilk

- 2 large eggs

- 3 cups mozzarella cheese (shredded)

- 4 ounces cream cheese

Instructions:

1. Preheat oven to 200 degrees C (400 degrees F). Line a baking tray with baking paper and set to one side

2. Melt the cream cheese and mozzarella cheese together in a small microwave bowl. Microwave at 1-minute intervals until the cheese begins to soften, then continue to microwave at 10 second intervals until the cheese has melted properly (be careful not to overcook)

3. Add the melted cheese and the remainder of your ingredients to a food processor. Pulse in the food processor until the ingredients have combined into a dough

4. Before handling the dough, grease your hands with a little oil to prevent it from sticking to you. This should make it easier to mold them into the right shapes

5. Take a handful of dough, roll it into a ball and place on a baking tray. While you can form them into any size you like, be wary about the cooking times – the larger the rolls are, the longer they will take to cook. The smaller they are, the faster they'll cook

6. Bake the rolls for between 13-18 minutes. When ready, they should be crusty on the outside and firm (but not hard) on the inside. Allow them to cool for at least 5 minutes before eating

7. Enjoy on their own with some butter, or as a side to one of our other low carb meals!

Hummus

Serves: 12 people

Prep Time: 10 minutes | Cook Time: 35 minutes | Total Time: 45 minutes

Calories: 109 | Net Carbs: 3g | Protein: 2g | Fat: 9g | Fiber: 1g

Ingredients:

- 1 ½ tsp cumin
- ½ cup (60g) tahini
- ¼ cup (60ml) Extra virgin olive oil
- ¼ tsp paprika
- 2 cloves of garlic (minced)
- 2 tbsp lemon juice
- 4 cups (520g) Cauliflower florets
- 4tbsp water
- Salt to taste

Instructions:

1. Preheat your oven to 400 degrees F (200 degrees C). Line a baking sheet with baking paper and set to one side

2. Coat the cauliflower florets with 2 tbsp of olive oil and spread across the baking sheet. spread them evenly and try not to have multiple pieces of cauliflower crowded on top of each other, because they won't cook evenly. If you need to, use multiple trays

3. Roast the cauliflower for around 40 minutes – make sure that it is browned and very soft. Cooking time is dependent on how large your pieces are. If you've cut the cauliflower quite small, it won't take as long

4. Pour the lemon juice, 2 tbsp water, 2 tbsp olive oil into a food processer. Add the rest of the ingredients and puree until it is very smooth. You may have to do this in short bursts and stop to scrape down the sides a couple of times

At-Home Guac

Serves: 4 people

Prep Time: 15 Minutes | Cook Time: 0 Minutes | Total Time: 15 Minutes

Calories: 234 | Net Carbs: 5g | Protein: 3g | Fat: 21g | Fiber: 8g

Ingredients:

- 1 garlic clove (minced)
- 1 tomato (diced)
- ½ a white onion (finely chopped)
- ¼ cup (4g) fresh coriander (cilantro)
- 2 large avocados
- 2 tbsp extra virgin olive oil
- Salt and pepper to your taste
- The juice of ½ a lime

Instructions:

1. Peel the avocados and de-pit them. Mash with a fork into a paste

2. Add the onion, lime juice, tomato, garlic and coriander, and mix well until all are combined

3. Season with salt and pepper to taste and serve – we like these with our seed crackers!

Sausage and egg grab and go muffins

Serves: 12 people

Prep Time: 20 minutes | Cook Time: 25 minutes | Total Time: 45 minutes

Calories: 98 | Net Carbs: 0.6g | Protein: 7.5g | Fat: 7g | Fiber: 0.4g

Ingredients:

- 1 cup (130g) cheddar cheese (shredded)
- 1 tbsp extra virgin olive oil
- ½ red bell pepper (diced)
- 10 regular eggs
- 1lb (600g) turkey sausage (ground)
- 2 tbsp fresh coriander (cilantro) (chopped)
- Salt and pepper, to taste

Instructions:

1. Preheat your oven to 350 degrees F, and preheat a frying pan or skillet over a medium heat

2. Grease 12 molds in a muffin tray and set to one side to be used later

3. Heat the olive oil in the pan, and then add the turkey sausage. Cook through until there is no pink remaining in the meat

4. Divide the cooked sausage evenly between the muffin tray molds. Also add a little of the cheese and red pepper to each of the molds

5. In a large mixing bowl, beat the eggs, salt, pepper and coriander, before pouring an even amount over each of the muffin molds. Sprinkle any of the remaining cheese over the top

6. Bake for 25 minutes until set. They should be golden on top, and firm throughout. Remove from the muffin tray and serve warm or allow to cool and then freeze to be reheated for later!

Seed crackers

Serves: 30 people

Prep Time: 15 Minutes | Cook Time: 45 Minutes | Total Time: 60 Minutes

Calories: 60 | Net Carbs: 1g | Protein: 2g | Fat: 6g | Fiber: 1g

Ingredients:

- 1 tbsp psyllium husk (ground into powder)
- ¼ tsp salt
- ¼ cup (60 ml) coconut oil (melted)
- 1 cup (240 ml) water (boiled)
- 1/3 cup (38g) almond flour
- 1/3 cup (45g) sunflower seeds
- 1/3 cup (45g) pumpkin seeds
- 1/3 cup (55g) black chia seeds

Instructions:

1. Preheat your oven to 300 degrees F (150 degrees C) and line a baking tray with baking paper. Set this to one side until needed later

2. In a mixing bowl, combine the dried ingredients and mix them together, before adding the boiling water and melted oil

3. Mix the water, oil and dried ingredients. While you stir, the chia seeds should start to soak up the water and form a gel – this is our dough

4. Put the chia and almond dough on the baking tray and press it out with your hands to flatten it. Then place a second sheet of baking paper over the chia and almond dough and use a rolling pin to flatten it across your baking sheet. Try to make it as even and flat as possible so that it bakes evenly

5. Remove the second sheet of paper and place in the oven on the middle shelf. Bake for about 40 minutes, checking occasionally. Be sure not to burn them

6. Turn off the oven, but don't remove the tray just yet. Leaving the tray inside while the oven cools will help to dry out the crackers. When dry (and cooled) break the sheet into pieces and serve – we recommend having them with our home made guac or hummus!

Energy Balls

Serves: 12 people

Prep Time: 10 minutes | Chill Time: 10 minutes | Total Time: 20 minutes

Calories: 140 | Net Carbs: 4.2g | Protein: 5.3g | Fat: 11.9g | Fiber: 3.3g

Ingredients:

- 1 cup (140g) sliced almonds
- 1 tbsp chia seeds
- ½ cup (20g) unsweetened natural peanut butter
- ¼ cup (15g) pumpkin seeds
- ¼ cup (20g) shredded coconut
- ¼ cup (45g) sugar free chocolate chips
- ¼ cup (80g) liquid sweetener
- 2 tbsp ground flaxseed

Instructions:

1. Add all the dried ingredients to a mixing bowl, stir them thoroughly and set the bowl aside. Line a plate with baking paper and also set to one side

2. Add the peanut butter and the liquid sweetener to a small microwave safe bowl. Microwave for 30 seconds to melt the two together, and then whisk together using a fork

3. Combine the liquid ingredients with the dried ingredients, using a spatula to stir them. This should form the ingredients into a sticky batter that can be molded

4. Before molding, grease your hands with a little coconut oil (or use a little butter), and roll out 12 energy balls. After each ball has been molded, feel free to roll them in extra sliced almonds or shredded coconut. Place each bowl on the plate you lined earlier

5. If you want to enjoy these straight away, put them in the freezer for 10 minutes to help firm them up. If not, then pack them into an airtight container in the fridge, where they'll keep for 2 weeks

Matthew Hollandar

Dessert Recipes

Blended Tofu Mousse

Serves: 4 people

Prep Time: 10 minutes | Chill Time: Overnight | Total Time: 12+ hours

Calories: 221 | Net Carbs: 2.1g | Protein: 14.3g | Fat: 16.3g | Fiber: 12.3g

Ingredients:

- 1 tbsp unsweetened cocoa powder (optional)
- 1 tsp coconut oil
- 1 tsp liquid sweetener
- 3 tbsp milk of choice (if you're using a dairy-free milk, make sure it's unsweetened, preferably almond)
- ¾ cup (100g) dark chocolate chips
- 400g silken tofu
- Pinch of salt

Instructions:

1. Add silken tofu, milk, liquid sweetener and salt to a blender. Blitz until combined into a smooth mixture

2. Use your microwave to melt the chocolate chips and coconut oil. Heat in increments of 30 seconds until completely melted (but avoid overheating)

3. Add the melted chocolate chips and coconut oil to the blender. Blend the mixture until completely smooth

4. Pour the mixture into 4 mason jars and seal tightly shut. Store in the fridge overnight to allow them to set

5. Before eating, sprinkle a little of the unsweetened cocoa powder over the top, and then enjoy!

Low Carb Cinnamon Rolls

Serves: 12 people

Prep Time: 35 minutes | Cook Time: 15 minutes | Total Time: 50 minutes

Calories: 183g | Net Carbs: 1g | Protein: 6g | Fat: 17g | Fiber: 2g

Ingredients:

For the dough

- 1 ½ cups (170g) mozzarella cheese (shredded)
- 1 cup (110g) almond flour
- 1 egg
- 1 tsp white wine vinegar
- ½ tsp baking powder
- ¼ cup (32g) powdered sweetener
- 2 tbsp coconut flour
- 2 tbsp cream cheese

For the filling

- 1 tbsp ground cinnamon
- ¼ cup (32g) powdered sweetener
- 4 oz (110g) butter (softened)

Matthew Hollandar

Instructions:

1. Preheat your oven to 365 degrees F (185 degrees C)

2. Add the mozzarella and cream cheese to a microwavable bowl and heat until the two have melted together. Remember to heat in small increments once you see the cheese begin to soften, because you don't want to overcook them. Alternatively, heat them in a pan on the stove

3. Add the flour, egg, ¼ cup powdered sweetener, baking powder and vinegar to the cheese and mix well until a dough is formed

4. Once you have your dough, roll it out over a sheet of baking paper to make a sheet about 3mm thick

5. In a small bowl, mix the cinnamon, powdered sweetener and softened (but not melted) butter together into a paste. Spread this evenly over the top of the dough

6. Using the baking paper, roll the dough tightly into a log. (Be careful not to get the paper caught in the layers of the log – roll it in the way you would roll sushi!)

7. Put it into the fridge to firm up the dough (this should take about 20 minutes)

8. Once the dough is firm, cut into 12 even pieces and place on a baking tray. Bake for about 10 minutes – until they are golden on top

9. Remove from the oven and allow to cool

10. If making an icing for the rolls, mix ¼ cup (32g) powdered sweetener and 1 tbsp of water together into a paste, and drizzle over the top

Matthew Hollandar

Vanilla Low Carb cake

Serves: 16 people

Prep Time: 15 minutes | Cook Time: 25 minutes | Total Time: 40 minutes

Calories: 172 | Net Carbs: 2g | Protein: 4g | Fat: 16g | Fiber: 3g

Ingredients:

- 1 ½ (cup 200g) almond flour
- 1 cup powdered sweetener
- 1 tsp vanilla extract
- ½ cup (120ml) almond milk
- ½ cup (70g) coconut flour
- ¼ tsp salt
- 2 tsp baking powder
- ¾ cup (100g) butter
- 4 large eggs
- Keto frosting of your choice (optional)

Instructions:

1. Preheat your oven to 350 degrees F (180 degrees C). Line 2 8-inch cake tins with baking paper and set to one side

2. In a large mixing bowl, add flower, baking powder and salt, and mix thoroughly

3. In a separate bowl, cream the butter and sweetener together until fluffy. One at a time, add the eggs and beat until they are fully mixed in

4. Add the milk and vanilla extract to the butter, and mix well

5. Add the dry ingredients a little bit at a time and beat well until a creamy batter forms. Be careful to make sure there are no lumps

6. Divide the batter evenly between the two cake tins and bake for around 24 minutes. When ready, the tops of the cakes should be golden, and a skewer should come out clean when stuck through the middle

7. Allow the cake to cool before frosting it with a keto-friendly frosting of your choice

Chia Seed Peanut Butter pudding

Serves: 2 people

Prep Time: 10 minutes | Chill Time: 30 Minutes | Total Time: 40 minutes

Calories: 162 | Net Carbs: 7.9g | Protein: 10.3g | Fat: 18g | Fiber: 12.1g

Ingredients:

- 1 ½ tbsp cocoa powder
- ½ cup (120ml) milk (if using dairy free milk choose an unsweetened kind, preferably almond)
- ½ cup whipped cream
- ½ tsp vanilla extract
- ¼ cup (30g) chia seeds
- 2 tbsp peanut butter
- 2 tbsp powdered sweetener

Instructions:

1. Combine all the ingredients except for the chia seeds in a large mixing bowl. Mix thoroughly with a whisk, taking care to whisk out any lumps from the cocoa powder Make sure to scrape the sides of the bowl to be sure that the peanut butter hasn't stuck to it

2. Whisk in the chia seeds, and then divide the mixture into 2 mason jars. Seal and put in the refrigerator to chill

3. Preferably chill the mixture overnight, but if you can't wait that long then at least chill for 30 minutes

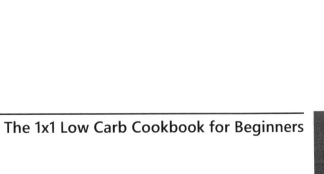

Disclaimer

This book contains opinions and ideas of the author and is meant to teach the reader informative and helpful knowledge while due care should be taken by the user in the application of the information provided. The instructions and strategies are possibly not right for every reader and there is no guarantee that they work for everyone. Using this book and implementing the information/recipes therein contained is explicitly your own responsibility and risk. This work with all its contents, does not guarantee correctness, completion, quality or correctness of the provided information. Misinformation or misprints cannot be completely eliminated.

Printed in Great Britain
by Amazon

80034913R00064